Ketogenic Diet and Lifestyle

Enjoy The Benefits of Keto Diet with this Essential and Complete Step by Step Beginner's Guide

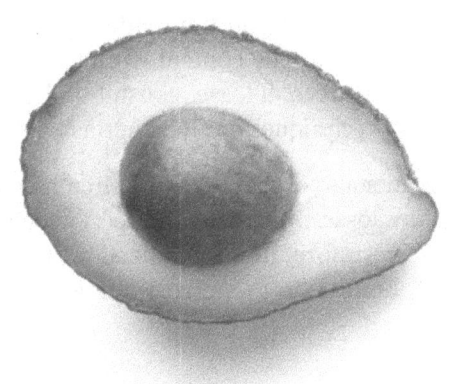

Dr. Suzanne Ramos Hughes, Amy Ryan

© Copyright 2021 - All rights reserved.

The content contained within this book may not be reproduced, duplicated or transmitted without direct written permission from the author or the publisher.

Under no circumstances will any blame or legal responsibility be held against the publisher, or author, for any damages, reparation, or monetary loss due to the information contained within this book. Either directly or indirectly.

Legal Notice:

This book is copyright protected. This book is only for personal use. You cannot amend, distribute, sell, use, quote or paraphrase any part, or the content within this book, without the consent of the author or publisher.

Disclaimer Notice:

Please note the information contained within this document is for educational and entertainment purposes only. All effort has been executed to present accurate, up to date, and reliable, complete information. No warranties of any kind are declared or implied. Readers acknowledge that the author is not engaging in the rendering of legal, financial, medical or professional advice. The content within this book has been derived from various sources. Please consult a licensed professional before attempting any techniques outlined in this book.

By reading this document, the reader agrees that under no circumstances is the author responsible for any losses, direct or indirect, which are incurred as a result of the use of information contained within this document, including, but not limited to, — errors, omissions, or inaccuracies.

Table of Contents

Introduction: The Beginner's Guide to a Better Life 1
Chapter 1: What the Ketogenic Diet Is 3
Chapter 2: Getting Started 11
Chapter 3: The Dos and Don'ts of the Keto Diet 19
Chapter 4: Why Keto? 27
Chapter 5: Cooking and Shopping 33
Chapter 6: Keto and Weight Loss FAQ 41
Chapter 7: Sample Meal Plan 47
Conclusion: Starting Your Keto Journey 55
References 59

Introduction:
The Beginner's Guide to a Better Life

These days, it seems like there are so many different kinds of trendy diets popping up from all parts of the globe. All of these diets come with their own pros and cons, but they all happen to have one thing in common - they help people maintain a healthier diet and lifestyle.

Among all of these trendy, modern diets, one of them stands out from all the rest, and that is the ketogenic diet. This diet has grown so popular that it's now considered a cultural craze. Of course, it wouldn't have become so famous unless it provided real benefits to actual people.

We all want to live a better life. However, most of the time we are so caught up with the hustle and bustle of our daily routine that we end up making food choices out of convenience instead of choosing options that are rich in the nutrients our bodies need. The good news is that you can change this part of your life any time you want to.

As long as you're willing to make the change and you've learned all that you can about the diet you plan to implement, the transition becomes smoother and easier, and that's exactly what you will be learning in this book. Here, you'll learn all about the ketogenic diet, such as how it works, how to begin using it, and so much more.

Chapter 1:
What the Ketogenic Diet Is

When it comes to learning about a new diet, you must always start with the basics. Unlike the many trendy or fad diets out there, the keto diet offers long-term success. This diet has been around since the 1920s, stemming from a solid understanding of nutrition science and physiology.

The keto diet is so successful because it targets the most common causes of weight gain, such as hormonal imbalances, insulin resistance, high levels of blood sugar, and the unending cycle of restricting one's food intake before binging on empty calories, an issue that a lot of people who want to lose weight struggle with. As a matter of fact, those are some of the most important results of this incredible diet.

So exactly what is the ketogenic diet?

The ketogenic, or "keto", diet doesn't mean counting your calories, limiting your portion sizes, or having to resort to extreme daily workout sessions. Rather, it's a low-carb diet that allows you to take a unique approach to health improvement and weight loss. One of the reasons why the keto diet works so well is that it changes your body's fuel source from burning sugar (glucose) to burning dietary fats.

When you start following this diet and you do it properly, your body will eventually reach a state known as "ketosis". When this happens, your body will begin burning up fats instead of sugar. If this is the first time you've really learned what the keto diet entails, you should also know that starting this diet is quite simple. Basically, you will need to do the following:

- Reduce your carb intake
- Eat more healthy fats to help you feel more sated

- Consume an approved list of foods that are specifically meant to help your body burn fats instead of sugars

Over time, the amount of glucose in your body diminishes which, in turn, forces your body to burn fat while producing ketones. As soon as your blood ketone level reaches a certain point, your body will reach ketosis. When you're in this state, you may experience rapid weight loss until you reach a weight that's both stable and healthy.

You can think of the keto diet as "tricking" your body into acting as if you're fasting as you eliminate the glucose from the carbs you were accustomed to eating in the past. The main aspect of this diet is to limit or restrict your intake of starch and sugar. When you consume these foods, your body breaks them down into sugar. When you eat too much, your body ends up storing these calories, thus they end up as body fat. Since the keto diet is a low-carb diet, this means that your body won't have any excess carbs to store. This is when it will start burning your fats in order to fuel your body each and every day.

How the Ketogenic Diet Works

The keto diet is all the rage right now. If you try searching for it on Google or another search engine, you'll discover a seemingly infinite amount of helpful and informative resources. Now that you understand what the keto diet involves, it's time to learn how it actually works. Knowing how the keto diet can benefit you will help you use it more effectively, and it will also help you understand why you need to follow the guidelines of the diet as religiously as possible.

The diet is high in fat, moderate in protein, and low in carbs. It's an eating pattern that strays from the standard healthful recommendations for eating. There are a lot of food items that are rich in nutrients but also rich in carbs, including whole grains, yogurt, milk, and some fruits and vegetables. When you're following the keto diet, you will have to stay away from these food items. Those who follow the diet try to consume less than 50 grams of carbs each day. Therefore, keto dieters don't eat cereals, bread, grains, or other types of high-carb food sources. Due to this restriction, starting the diet results in a huge shift in how most people typically eat.

Carbohydrates are your body's primary energy source. When you restrict this macronutrient from your body, it won't have enough fuel for energy; therefore, your body will start breaking down fats into ketones, and then the ketones become your body's main fuel source. They provide the energy needed by the kidneys, heart, and all of the other organs and muscles. Also, the body will start using the ketones it produces as the brain's energy source.

The keto diet serves as a partial fast for the body. When you fast completely or when you're in a state of starvation, your body doesn't have an energy source. Therefore, it starts breaking down your lean muscle mass to keep it going. Since the keto diet doesn't involve starvation or complete fasting, your body will be able to maintain its lean muscle mass as it targets the fats.

As popular as this diet is, it remains highly controversial, mainly because it involves consuming high amounts of fat. Several studies have shown that high-fat diets might increase the risk of chronic diseases such as heart disease. This is why it's highly recommended that you consult with your doctor first before starting the keto diet. It's important to keep in mind that you must follow the diet correctly if you really want to enjoy all the benefits without having to worry about the risks.

One more thing to try to remember when it comes to the keto diet is that individual BMI and metabolic rates of each person have an effect on how quickly their bodies are able to produce ketones. This explains why some people lose weight a lot faster than others, even when starting the keto diet at the same time. This is also the reason why some people give up too quickly; they don't see the results as early as they would like.

The bottom line is that the keto diet is quite restrictive and it does come with its own risks, but this is true for any type of diet. However, the great thing about the keto diet is that it has been around for quite some time now, and through the years, it has been refined and modified in order to help produce all the benefits people are looking for. So if you want to make your life better, the keto diet may be the best way to begin doing so.

A Short History

Although you may have already heard about the incredible weight loss benefits of the keto diet, it wasn't actually developed for this purpose alone. People have been using fasting as part of a treatment for epilepsy since as early as 500 BC. In the case of the keto diet, you are avoiding glucose. Normally, our bodies run on sugars derived from the carbohydrates we consume. Typically, our muscles and liver store up to 2,000 calories worth of sugar, and the body is able to burn through this stored sugar in about two days. After this time, when there's no sugar left due to avoiding carbs, the body starts burning its stored fat.

Back in the early part of the 1920s, one of the doctors of the Mayo Clinic, Dr. Russel Wilder, MD, began developing the keto diet which, back then, was nothing more than a fat-centered diet that replicated the effects of fasting through the depletion of sugar in the body. After developing the diet, Dr. Wilder tested it on those who suffered from epilepsy and found out how effective it was. Since then, it has been used as part of a treatment for seizures.

The main concept behind the keto diet is very simple. People can remain in an indefinite fasting state as long as they limit or eliminate carbs from their diet. This causes their bodies to burn fat rather than glucose. This shift in the dietary ratio in favor of fat eliminated sugar, thus triggering the body to function using ketones instead. Simply put, following this diet convinces the body to act the same way as if it were starving after consuming enough nutrition and calories to remain healthy.

Dr. Peterman, another doctor from the Mayo Clinic, termed this diet as the "keto approach", which still exists today. In this classic approach, it's recommended to consume specific types of foods in order to keep the body going while also cutting down your consumption of carbohydrates, sugars, and starches. As effective as this diet was, it was only seen as part of a treatment for epilepsy.

However, as more and more anticonvulsant medications were developed, this diet lost its place in the limelight.

So, why is it so popular now?

Much of the credit for the re-emergence of this diet goes to the TV show "Dateline". One particular episode that aired back in October of 1994 focused on the life of a two-year-old child named Charlie, who suffered from severe epilepsy. After starting the keto diet, Charlie's seizures began to diminish. As everyone watched little Charlie get better as a result of the keto diet, scientists started becoming interested in it once again, though still primarily as a treatment for epilepsy. Although people with epilepsy aren't the only ones who follow this diet.

Though it isn't entirely clear when people started experiencing the weight loss benefits of this diet, it may have begun around the late 90s when other low-carb diets were also very popular. Diets such as Atkins caused researchers to have a renewed interest in the keto diet, and through their research, they discovered some impressive results. Nowadays, people follow the keto diet for weight loss, as well as for other health reasons.

Success Stories

It's one thing to know the definition and history of a specific diet, but it's another thing to hear what real people have to say about it. So many people have started following this diet and very few of them have quit, especially after they started experiencing the many benefits of the keto diet. This diet has become so popular all over the world that it has a loyal following. Before we delve into the many benefits of the keto diet, let's take a look at some success stories from those who have actually reached their health goals because of it.

1. **Emily from Miami, Florida**

    For years, Emily was eating herself into an early grave, but when she was informed of how close she was to developing a serious heart condition, it served as her wakeup call. When she began using the keto diet, she was able to shed enough weight in a matter of 8 months so as to no longer fall under the "morbidly obese" category.

2. **Emma from London, United Kingdom**

    Emma's job required her to work 80 hours a week, plus 10 hours total for commuting, which didn't leave much room for regular exercise and health-conscious eating. She felt like her lifestyle was killing her slowly; that is, until she discovered the ketogenic diet. Although she still isn't able to exercise regularly, she can follow this diet because of how simple and mainstream it is. She also has noticed that she has a lot more energy, making her more productive at her job.

3. **Jake from Perth, Australia**

    Jake learned about the keto diet as he was searching for natural remedies for his mental health issues. For him, anxiety was a crippling aspect of his life. Although the medications he was taking helped out, he didn't want to become dependent on them. When his dietitian recommended the keto diet, he started following it. His mental health has improved so much that his anxiety attacks are now a rare occurrence.

4. **Jason from San Diego, California**

    Jason has been a fan of this diet since his doctor recommended it as a way to help him manage his diabetes. In his first year, Jason lost more than 20 pounds. Through this diet, he's able to maintain a healthy weight without having to rely on medications to manage his condition.

5. **Kate from Ontario, Canada**

    Kate started on keto about 6 months ago, and according to her, the diet has improved all aspects of her life. Her goal was to shed 20 pounds, but in total, she lost 25 pounds. She followed the keto diet and paired it with regular exercise, both of which helped her break her unhealthy habits.

6. **Sandra from Singapore**

Sandra saw how the keto diet had drastically improved her husband's life when he started on it as a way to help his diabetes. She started trying out her husband's keto snacks and realized that she would be able to follow this kind of diet herself. Since then, she has lost a good amount of weight while feeling more active and healthier.

7. **Tony from Albany, New York**

Although type 2 diabetes runs in his family, Tony couldn't seem to kick his fast foods and sugar addictions. What opened his eyes was when he experienced a mild heart attack at 45 years of age. He knew that he had to lose weight, and when he learned about the keto diet, it made a lot of sense to him. As soon as he started, he just kept going. He has been on this diet for more than 2 years now, and he just completed his very first marathon.

Those are just a few examples of success stories shared by real people this year. Imagine how many more around the world have their own success stories to share. Also, imagine how much the keto diet can change your life once you begin using it and following it properly. When it comes to keto, the possibilities for improvement are endless.

Chapter 2: Getting Started

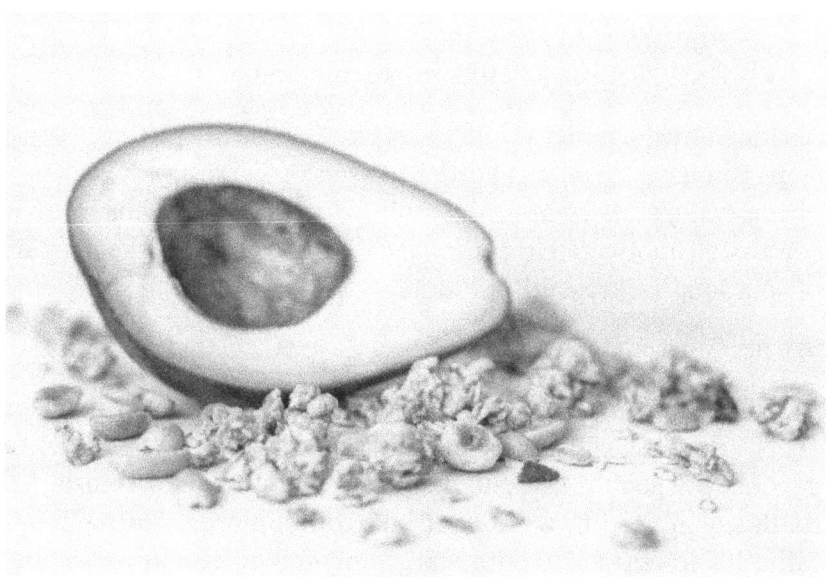

Learning all about the keto diet is just the first step of your journey. By now, you may already want to start modifying your diet so that you can enjoy all the benefits of this healthy way of eating. Keep in mind, though, that changing your diet is not a simple task, especially if you are currently eating whatever you want regardless of how greasy, loaded with carbs, and unhealthy the food is. Part of getting started is making the decision to learn everything that you can about it so that you can follow the diet properly.

Unlike other diets out there, the keto diet is fairly restrictive. You should prepare yourself for this fact so you don't end up regretting your decision; just like any other diet, the longer you stick with it, the easier it gets. After some time, you will start experiencing the many health benefits which, hopefully, will help keep you motivated. In terms of getting started, some important steps include the following:

- Know exactly which type of foods you can eat and which ones you should avoid.
- Learn how to figure out and keep track of your macros.
- Plan your meals each day so that you can reach ketosis quickly.
- Keep testing your ketones so you know when to make adjustments to your diet.
- Reach ketosis and then try to maintain it.

Although the keto diet is more elaborate, these are the most basic steps you have to follow in order to use the diet properly. Outside of these steps, there are many things you can do to ensure that you're well-motivated to continue with the diet and make it a part of your long-term health solution.

Setting Goals and Planning

After making the decision to go keto, it's time to start setting your goals, and these will be the foundation for the plans you make. In general, the goal of the keto diet is to reach a state of ketosis. To do this, you need to wean your body off of glucose for the long-term. It's important to note that simply following a low-carb diet won't guarantee that you will achieve ketosis. For some low-carb diets, you may enter ketosis for a while, but you can go back to burning glucose once you've returned to your old eating habits.

This is where the ketogenic diet stands out from the rest. It's more of a medical diet that has been developed with careful precision to ensure that you will reach ketosis and stay there in order to experience all of the long-term health benefits of doing so. The good news is that there are different types of keto diets to choose from. Base your choice on your current fitness level, your health goals, and what is realistic for your own lifestyle.

The different keto diets are provided below:

- **Standard Ketogenic Diet (SKD)**
  This is the most recommended and most commonly followed type of keto diet. While following the SKD, you should only consume between 20-50 grams of carbs each

day. Also, you need to focus on high-fat and moderate-protein intake.

- **Targeted Ketogenic Diet (TKD)**
  This type of keto diet is most recommended for those who have a very active lifestyle. While following this diet, you must only consume between 25-50 grams of carbs. You also need to make sure to consume these carbs less than half an hour to one hour before you work out.

- **Cyclical Ketogenic Diet (CKD)**
  If you want to follow the keto diet but it seems a bit intimidating to you, then it may be best to start with this type. While following the CKD, you cycle between periods of consuming a low-carb diet for a certain number of days followed by a period of eating a moderate amount of carbs for a certain number of days. You can continue doing this until you're more comfortable with following the SKD or any other type of keto diet more permanently.

- **High Protein Ketogenic Diet (HPKD)**
  This type of keto diet is a lot like the SKD. The main difference is that you consume more than moderate amounts of protein.

- **Plant-Based Ketogenic Diet (PBKD)**
  Finally, this type of keto diet may range from simply eating more veggies that are low in carbs to following the keto diet as a full-on vegetarian or vegan. If you choose the latter, prepare yourself to put in a lot of effort and work into your diet to ensure that you follow it correctly and safely.

After determining which type of keto diet you would like to follow, it's time to set your goals. Make sure that you set a goal that's "SMART" or specific, measurable, attainable, realistic, and time-bound. You may think of this goal as your map which leads you to your intended destination. When thinking of your main health goal, you might want to try answering these questions:

- Would you like to live healthier in the long-run?

- Would you like to reduce your dependency on medications?
- Would you like to manage your diabetes more effectively?
- Would you like to lose weight?

These are some excellent questions that can guide you as you think about your goal. No matter what goal you come up with, you will be able to achieve this through planning and by taking things one day and one step at a time.

Let's look at an example to better illustrate the use of SMART goals for your keto diet:

- **Goal:** Weight loss
- **Specific:** I would like to lose 3 pounds each month by limiting myself to consuming less than 25 grams of carbs each day.
- **Measurable:** I will measure my weight on the same day each month to see how I am progressing.
- **Attainable:** I will only consume the foods that are recommended for the SKD.
- **Realistic:** I will drink more water each day rather than drinking beverages that have sugar content.
- **Time-Bound:** I would like to lose up to 18 pounds after 6 months by following the steps and plans I have made.

As you can see, you have a main goal and a few smaller goals that are easier to achieve. Each time you achieve these smaller goals, you get closer and closer to your main goal. This is just one example of how you can set your goals and plan how to achieve them. You can make your own plans according to your health and fitness goals.

The Most Common Keto-Friendly Ingredients

With all of the health benefits the ketogenic diet offers, it almost seems like a dream come true. Imagine - you're encouraged to eat a lot of cheese, meat, nuts, dressing, and so on, but on the other side of the coin, you should also be very careful when it comes to your carb intake. There are a lot of whole grains, veggies, fruits, and more that you would need to stop eating no matter how much you love them. Otherwise, you might end up gaining weight instead of losing it.

As you will discover later on, a huge part of being able to stick with the keto lifestyle is learning how to cook keto-friendly meals. This is especially true if you live in areas where there aren't a lot of ready-to-eat food options that fit into your diet. If you plan to cook your meals, you must know which ingredients are keto-friendly. Let's take a look at the most common ones:

- **Condiments**

  Most condiments are keto-friendly. For some options, though, you may need to make a couple of minor adjustments. Also, check the labels of the condiments you purchase to make sure they don't contain any added sugar. While following the keto diet, you may use condiments such as the following:

  - Mayonnaise
  - Ketchup
  - Buffalo sauce
  - Salad dressings

- **Oils**

  The keto diet focuses on consuming a lot of fats, especially the healthy types of fats. This is why you have quite a lot of options when it comes to oils. Some of the more common ones used for cooking include:

  - Medium-chain triglycerides, or MCT, oil
  - Coconut oil
  - Cooking oil like sunflower seed oil, avocado oil, grapeseed oil, and others
  - Non-cooking oil like pistachio oil, walnut oil, flaxseed oil, and others

- **Ghee**

  Although this is against most kinds of diets, butter is a welcome addition to the keto diet, so go ahead and use it while cooking. Clarified butter, or ghee, is also encouraged, and it will impart a rich nuttiness to your dishes that you won't get from butter.

- **Seeds and nuts**
  Most types of nuts are excellent sources of healthy fats. They also have a lot of fiber. However, some nuts may contain more carbs than others, so make sure to do your research before snacking on these or adding them to your cooking. As for seeds, you can add them to your snacks and blended smoothies and sprinkle them over your salads.

- **Nut butters**
  Most peanut butter products contain added sugar, so when you're on the keto diet, you should opt for unsweetened varieties. Apart from peanut butter, you have other options as well, such as almond butter, cashew butter, walnut butter, and so on. You can use these for different dishes as long as you choose the unsweetened varieties.

- **Keto-friendly sweeteners**
  Although a lot of keto dieters prefer to avoid sweeteners altogether, for some this can be quite difficult, especially at the beginning. If you're one such person, you can choose to use keto-friendly sweeteners in your recipes. Some examples of these include sucralose, erythritol, monk fruit, and stevia. However, you may also want to search for keto-friendly recipes that use these types of sweeteners to ensure that they work well.

- **Thickeners and flours**
  You don't have to give up baked goods when you follow this diet. However, you will have to modify the ingredients you use for your recipes. Some keto-friendly flours include almond meal, coconut flour, almond flour, and others. You can also use these keto-friendly options for thickening stews, sauces, and soups.

- **Salt**
  When it comes to the keto diet, you need to include salt. This is an important ingredient as it can help ease the occurrence of electrolyte swings. Apart from normal salt, you can include some flavored salts to your arsenal to enhance the taste of your dishes.

Finding Support

Some people have a difficult time finding the motivation they need within themselves to stick with the keto diet. In such cases, finding support is crucial. In any new venture, having a great support system can undoubtedly help you succeed. Remember that the keto diet is quite different from traditional diets. Therefore, you may experience some changes in your body that might make you feel apprehensive, especially at the beginning.

As we have established, the keto diet is already quite famous all around the world. This means that there is a high likelihood of being able to find support, even in the most unexpected places. You can ask people at work, your friends, and your family members for support. Maybe some of them have already been following the keto diet and have some advice to share with you.

Some of the more common issues experienced by those who start the keto diet include:

- Adjusting to consuming fewer carbs each day
- Developing a condition known as the keto flu
- Experiencing new feelings and sensations caused by the diet change
- Craving high-carb foods that you're used to eating
- Not losing weight right away

If you experience any of these issues or any other issues related to your diet, you may want to seek out support. We've shared some success stories in the previous chapter; if you search online, you will be able to read a lot more of these stories. There are also a lot of online forums and support groups that you can join to have conversations with people and ask for advice from the other members. No matter where you find your support, doing so will surely help you stick with your diet for the long haul.

Chapter 3:
The Dos and Don'ts of the Keto Diet

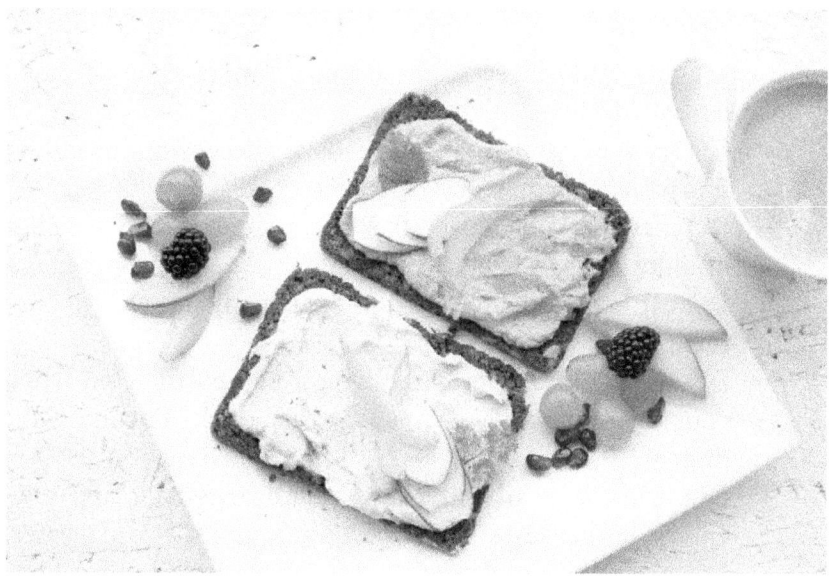

After setting your goals and coming up with a plan to reach those goals, it's time to start learning more about the keto diet, specifically the dos and don'ts of this high-fat, low-carb diet. The keto diet can help you lose weight and feel better as long as you follow all the commands, guidelines, and recommendations. The diet comes with quite a lot of rules, but fortunately, they're easy to follow.

Conversely, if you don't go keto the correct way, you shouldn't expect to experience all of the benefits you're aiming for. Just like any other diet, properly following it is key. The more you adhere to the rules and guidelines of the keto diet, the higher the likelihood of reaching your health and fitness goals. With that being said, let's begin by discussing what you should be doing.

Do These Things on the Keto Diet

When it comes to the dos of the keto diet, what is most important is paying attention to the types of food you eat. Later on, we will go over a more detailed list of these foods; however, for now, let's take a look at the general guidelines to follow after going keto:

- DO eat a lot of leafy greens, such as cabbage, kale, spinach, arugula, and others, as these contain minimal amounts of carbohydrates.
- DO increase your intake of seeds as these contain healthy fats which can help you reach ketogenesis faster.
- DO increase your nut intake, either as part of your dishes or enjoyed as a snack.
- DO eat lean proteins, such as eggs, fish, and lean cuts of meat.
- DO use high-fat oils like olive oil and coconut oil when cooking as an easy way to add more healthy fats into your diet.
- DO drink a lot of water along with low-sugar and low-calorie beverages, such as tea, coffee, and sparkling water.
- DO eat more "real foods" instead of processed or pre-packaged foods.
- DO maintain healthy levels of electrolytes in your body by drinking chicken or bone broth seasoned with salt.
- DO make use of natural, keto free sweeteners when you really need your sugar fix.
- DO try to stay away from fast foods as these typically contain a lot of unhealthy and high-carb ingredients.
- DO make sure that you eat three meals each day regularly plus keto-friendly snacks in between when you're feeling hungry.
- DO add around 2 teaspoons of salt to your daily diet to help you feel better.
- DO add around 3-4 tablespoons of fat to each of your meals as the keto diet is high in fat.
- DO pair your keto diet with regular exercise to remain healthy and active throughout the day.

- DO get enough sleep so your body will be able to manage stress more effectively.
- DO make sure that your plate contains veggies at every meal, including breakfast.
- DO stop eating as soon as you feel full.
- DO remind yourself why you started the diet in the first place in order to keep yourself motivated.

Don't Do These Things on the Keto Diet

Of course, there is always the other side of the coin. While there are things you must do while following the keto diet, there are also things which you must avoid. Keep these in mind if you want to be able to go keto in the most effective way:

- DON'T eat fruits that are high in sugar and carbohydrates, such as bananas, grapes, mangoes, cherries, and others.
- DON'T buy food items that are grain-based, such as cookies, pasta, rice, and bread, as these typically contain high amounts of starch, calories, and carbs.
- DON'T consume sugar, whether in its natural or processed form.
- DON'T eat vegetables that are high in carbs, such as corn, sweet potatoes, white potatoes, and the like.
- DON'T drink beverages high in calories and sugar.
- DON'T eat more carbs than what's recommended since the keto diet is mainly focused on reducing your carb intake to the bare minimum.
- DON'T eat "low-carb" or "sugar-free" processed foods as these typically contain unwanted calories and ingredients.
- DON'T eat "low-fat" foods since the keto diet focuses on consuming high amounts of fats.
- DON'T eat bad fats that you typically get from canola oil, vegetable oil, corn oil, hydrogenated oil, and soybean oil
- DON'T check the labels of the foods you eat after eating them; always check the labels before putting anything in your mouth.
- DON'T obsess over your macros; just keep track of them and make yourself aware of how your body is feeling.

- DON'T worry if you have a slip up once in a while as long as you get right back on track afterward.
- DON'T tell yourself you'll only have a bite every so often just so you can taste the foods you're craving but that aren't recommended on the keto diet.
- DON'T test your ketone and blood glucose levels more than two times a day unless your doctor recommends it.
- DON'T forget to take supplements if you or your doctor think you need them.
- DON'T forget to praise and encourage yourself after each day you've managed to remain on the keto diet without slipping up.

Maintaining a Positive Attitude

The longer you stick with the keto diet, the more you'll learn about it, and once you start experiencing all of the health benefits, the more motivated you will become. If you're just starting your keto journey, maintaining a positive attitude will help you out tremendously. Believing in the diet and in how it can potentially improve your life in the long-term will have a huge impact on how successful you are at following it.

As popular and beneficial as this diet may be, it can still be quite challenging to follow, especially if you are a lover of sugary and carb-rich foods. There also exists the possibility of getting the keto flu, which happens to some people. So how do you maintain the positive attitude required to keep going?

Here are some tips that may help to guide you:

- **When it comes to meal planning, don't take things too seriously** - Meal planning is an important part of the keto diet, especially if you really want to stick with keto-friendly meals each and every time. However, just because you've made plans doesn't mean you should restrict yourself too much. If you have a meal planned for lunch and you're either not hungry or you're craving something else, place that planned meal back in the refrigerator and eat what you're craving (as long as it's also keto-friendly).

- **Listen to your body** - This is one of the most important things you must do, especially during the beginning of your keto journey. You should never push yourself so hard that you end up getting sick or feeling miserable. Part of the change is to feel comfortable with this new diet, and the best way for you to do this is by listening to yourself and being mindful of your body.
- **Learn more about your favorite foods and which ones you can still eat while following the keto diet** - This is a great way to stay positive, especially if a lot of your favorite foods make the list. From your favorite fruits, vegetables, proteins, and even fat sources, learning more about different types of food helps you stay on track.
- **Know the risks** - If you don't suffer from any medical conditions and you just want to start a healthier diet, then all you have to do is learn all you can about keto, including the risks. However, if you suffer from any kind of medical condition or you're taking medication(s), then you must first consult with your doctor about the idea of starting keto. This will help you avoid any unexpected drawbacks that might cause you to give up.
- **Always do what is best for you and your health** - Finally, when it comes to going keto (or starting any other kind of diet, for that matter), you must always think about your own health and safety. Never sacrifice either of these just to reach your health goals. It's better to experience a gradual transition that provides long-term benefits than a quick change that does more harm than good.

Coping with the Adjustment

For some people, starting the keto diet can be very challenging, but this doesn't make keto an impossible quest. Just as with any other major lifestyle change, it does take time and effort to adjust to this novel way of eating. Fortunately, as long as you have enough information, helpful tips, and useful strategies, you will be able to cope with the adjustment.

To help ease your journey, here are some things to keep in mind:

- **Learn how to differentiate keto-friendly and non-keto foods** - This is probably one of the most challenging things people have to deal with on the keto diet. Since there are some types of foods that you should avoid while following this diet, you must be able to differentiate between them. To do this, you must understand the type of keto diet you're following and what it entails. As long as you know how much of each macronutrient you must consume each day, knowing what you can eat becomes a lot easier. Then, all you have to do is read food labels to determine whether or not what you're about to purchase or consume is keto-friendly.
- **Learn how to calculate your net carb intake** - The main restriction on the keto diet is your carb intake. Unless you follow this golden rule, you won't be able to reach ketosis. Therefore, learning how to calculate your net carbs will help you determine when you've had enough for the day so you can find other types of food to eat.
- **Create a keto-friendly food environment** - This is a lot easier if you live on your own. All you have to do is clean up your kitchen and stock up on keto-friendly foods. However, when you live with other people in your home, then you should speak to them about your lifestyle change, and then you can create your own "keto-corner" in your kitchen or pantry to ensure that you always have your own food to snack on or your own ingredients to cook when necessary.
- **Be mindful of everything you're eating** - Finally, learn how to be mindful of everything you're eating. Gone are the days of simply picking up whatever's available and eating it just because you're in a rush and it's more convenient. If you really want to stick with this diet, it's time to make yourself more aware of what you're putting into your body. Over time, learning which foods are allowed and which ones you should avoid become easier,

making it less challenging for you to cope with the diet and focus on other things.

Chapter 4:
Why Keto?

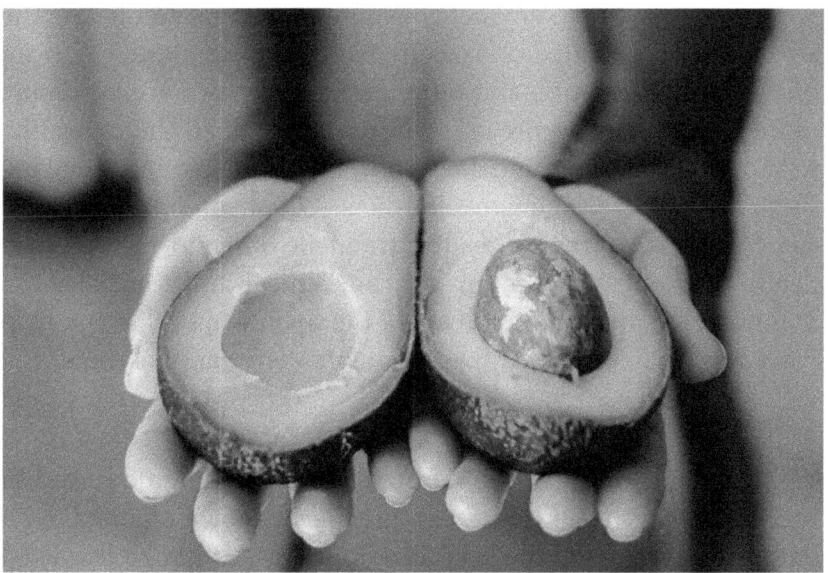

If you're thinking about starting a new diet and you try doing an online search, you will come up with various kinds of diets that claim to be the best ones; this can make you feel overwhelmed. So you may ask yourself why you should choose keto. What makes this diet stand out from all the others?

Let's say you've already tried one of the trendy diets out there. However, even though you've followed all the rules, you're still not able to reach your health and fitness goals; or because of the diet, your health suffers, and your doctor recommends to put you on medications; or you're trying to overcome or better manage a condition through your diet, but it just isn't happening. How can you start making your life better?

Of course, starting a healthy diet is the first step, but when you're trying to lose weight or dealing with medical conditions, you should pick the right diet to suit your own needs. Although there is no single diet that works for everyone, the standard ketogenic diet, or SKD, does have a lot of evidence supporting its health benefits. There are also a lot of anecdotal reports and success stories from real people claiming how effective this diet has been for them.

At the very core, the keto diet goes a long way into combating the adverse effects created or exacerbated by the standard American diet. Diabetes, obesity, and other chronic diseases are becoming more and more widespread, mainly because of all the unhealthy food options out there and due to how liberal people are at making these foods part of their regular diets. When you opt for keto, it can help reverse the unhealthy trend in order to restore your health without the use of pharmaceutical interventions. As mentioned earlier, keto is a type of therapeutic diet that can help you embrace foods that will adequately satisfy and fuel you.

The Benefits of the Keto Diet

The ketogenic diet has been around for some time now, and in recent years, it has become very popularly known among health enthusiasts as one of the best diets to follow. Although it started out as part of a treatment for epilepsy, research and studies have shown that the benefits of this diet go beyond reducing the occurrence of seizures. If you're planning to go keto, here are some benefits you can look forward to:

- **Reduced inflammation** - The ability to drastically reduce inflammation in the body is one of the most fundamental and significant benefits of the keto diet. This happens because of the reduced production of free radicals when the body burns ketones for fuel rather than glucose. Reduced inflammation allows your body to produce more energy which, in turn, helps you function more efficiently.
- **Improved fat burning** - This is one of the most popular benefits of this diet, especially for those who would like to lose weight. When you reach ketosis, it means that your body is burning fat for fuel. Therefore, if you're struggling

with excess body fat, you will be able to get rid of it at a faster and more efficient rate.

- **Mental sharpness and clarity** - After some time, you may start noticing that your mind is a lot sharper and clearer. This is due to the reduction of neurological inflammation which is associated with poor cognitive functions, anxiety, and depression.

- **More energy** - This benefit comes from the fact that you have stable blood sugar levels, reduced inflammation, upregulation of mitochondrial biogenesis, and more ATP for each molecule of ketones. All of these benefits combined have a significant impact on your energy levels, allowing you to stay active and productive all throughout the day.

- **Clearer and smoother skin** - There are a lot of skin conditions, such as acne, psoriasis, eczema, and others, that are caused by autoimmunity or chronic inflammation. Since following the keto diet helps reduce inflammation, it may be beneficial to your skin health.

- **Reduced cravings** - The longer you stick with the diet, the more you will notice that you don't crave those high-carb and high-sugar foods anymore. Your body will start getting used to your new diet, allowing you to eat healthier without having to focus on the foods that may prevent you from maintaining a state of ketogenesis.

- **Anti-aging** - This benefit is also connected to the reduced production of free radicals. These free radicals play an important role in the aging process wherein they make you age a lot faster, but since your body will be running on ketones instead of glucose, it won't produce large amounts of these free radicals. Therefore, you may notice that the aging process doesn't seem to affect you as quickly as it did before.

These are some of the general benefits of the keto diet that apply to healthy individuals. Of course, if you're suffering from a medical condition and your doctor recommends that you go keto, it's because this diet has a lot of medical-related benefits as well. The bottom line is that the keto diet comes with several long-term benefits to ensure that you will live a long, happy, and healthy life.

Combining Keto with Other Wellness Techniques

Speaking of benefits, another great thing about the keto diet is that you don't have to follow it exclusively. On its own, it's amazing, but you can also combine it with other wellness techniques or diets in order to enhance its effects and help you reach your goals faster. Let's take a look at the most commonly used combinations involving the keto diet.

Keto and Intermittent Fasting

The ketogenic diet and intermittent fasting are the hottest health trends right now. A lot of health enthusiasts use these diets to reach their goals of losing weight or managing their health conditions. Both diets come with their own pros that outweigh the cons.

By now, you already know quite a lot about the keto diet, so let's discuss intermittent fasting. Basically, this is a type of eating method where you cycle between fasting (calorie restriction) and normal consumption of food during a certain period of time. One thing it has in common with keto is that it has several types or variations. Although most people follow this diet mainly for weight loss, it does offer a number of health benefits.

We've already established how effective and beneficial the keto diet is, so why combine it with intermittent fasting? Combining both diets may help you achieve ketosis a lot more quickly than when you only follow the keto diet. The reason for this is that when you're fasting, the body maintains its balance of energy by using fats as its fuel source (since you limit your carb and sugar intake).

Combining both diets may also result in more fat loss. Since keto helps you lose weight and intermittent fasting also helps you lose weight, combining the two speeds up the process significantly.

Following both diets simultaneously is quite safe for most people. However, if you're pregnant, breastfeeding, or if you suffer from any kind of eating disorder, it's not recommended for you to do this. Also, if you have any kind of medical condition, consult with your doctor first to find out if it's advisable for you to combine these diets.

Keto and the Paleo Diet

Have you ever tried doing an online search for the keto diet? You may have noticed how keto is frequently compared with paleo, even though the two diets are very different. For the paleo diet, you are required to eat real, whole foods, just like the cavemen in the past. You focus on meat, fish, vegetables, fruits, seeds, and nuts. Here, you don't have to watch your carb intake as long as you're eating foods that people used to eat during the Paleolithic era.

This is another diet that may work well with keto to provide you with more mental clarity, help you lose weight faster, and give you more energy. Combining these two diets may work wonders for a few reasons.

Their combination allows you to control your appetite more effectively which, in turn, helps you lose weight faster. Also, combining both diets helps reduce the risk of developing cardiovascular diseases by lowering the levels of bad cholesterol, and they can also help you sleep better each night, in turn, strengthening your immune system.

Before combining keto with paleo or any other kind of diet or wellness technique, it's important for you to learn everything you can about the proper way to do this, as well as the risks involved and the potential benefits. Consulting with your doctor is crucial in order to ensure your long-term health and safety.

Chapter 5:
Cooking and Shopping

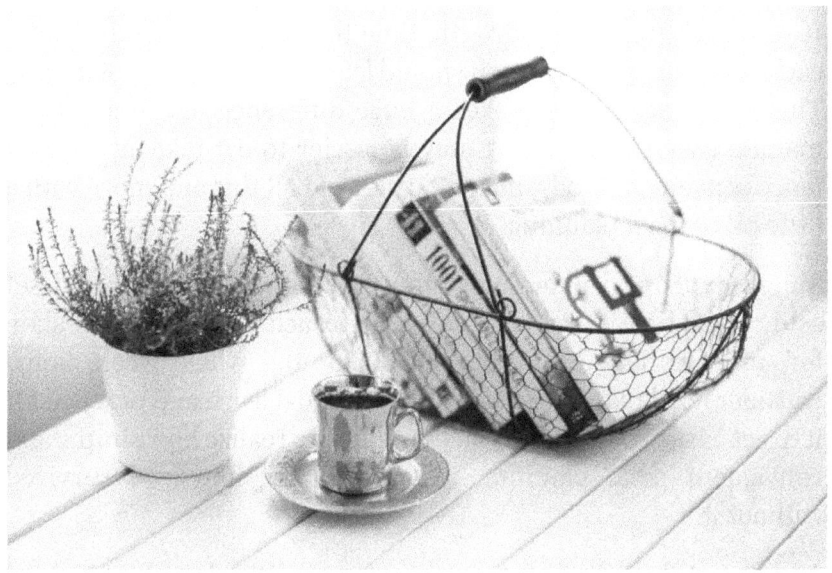

Cooking is a huge part of the keto diet. If you love cooking, then starting your keto journey can be a whole lot easier and more interesting for you. If you're not really a fan of cooking or preparing your own meals, it's time to start learning.

One of the main reasons that cooking is an important part of the keto diet is that it helps you stick with your diet better. Most people end up eating unhealthy foods and meals because they choose the convenient options. Unfortunately, those convenient options also happen to be extremely unhealthy. Many pre-packaged, processed, and ready-to-eat meals typically contain added ingredients and calories that aren't allowed on the keto diet, either.

So the best thing for you to do is to start cooking your own meals. There may be a good amount of keto-friendly options available now compared to a few years ago, but cooking your own meals is still the healthier and more economical way to go. If you start cooking your own food, then you must learn how to shop for all the best keto ingredients. Cooking and shopping go hand-in-hand, which is why there is one whole chapter dedicated to these tasks.

All About Meal Planning

If you don't think you have the time to cook keto-friendly meals each and every day, then you should learn all about meal planning. This is a process that makes a huge difference in the ability to maintain your new diet. It may be easier to eat takeout or cook more convenient foods, but you can avoid all this and more with a little bit of meal planning.

Simply put, meal planning is the process where you would set aside some time - such as a day or two each week - to plan, shop for, prepare, and cook your meals for the whole week. Some consider meal planning a skill that you must learn and practice for it to get easier. Over time, you may come to realize how simple and convenient meal planning is and wonder how you survived without it.

Are you still in doubt? Here are some of the benefits of meal planning that you can look forward to:

- **It's economical** - While a lot of people believe that going keto is expensive, this doesn't have to be the case - that is, if you start meal planning. This process involves shopping for fresh ingredients to whip up different dishes. Raw ingredients are a lot cheaper than prepared meals, which means that, in the long run, you'll be saving a lot of money.

- **You can eat real food** - The keto diet comes with several food rules that you must adhere to if you want it to be effective. How can you do this when you eat meals that have been prepared by other people? When you practice meal planning, you will be cooking your own meals, allowing you to choose what goes into your dishes. This means that you are sure that what you're eating is real food and that everything you eat fits in with your diet.

- **It helps reduce food waste** - Meal planning allows you to control your portion sizes. You can pack your meals according to how much you can actually eat. This means that you won't have any leftovers or food waste, unlike when you dine out and you're served with huge portions that you can't finish in one sitting.

- **It makes you feel less stressed** - If you don't want to feel stressed because you can't find keto-friendly food options in restaurants, your office cafeteria, or at other food establishments, then you should definitely start meal planning. This allows you to have your own meals ready for consumption whether or not there are any other options available.

- **It saves you time** - You don't have to spend time cooking before each meal. Remember, meal planning involves setting a schedule to prepare and cook all of your meals for the week. Once you've gotten the hang of meal planning, you'll be able to do it much faster. When you're ready to eat, all you have to do is take your meal from the refrigerator, heat it up if necessary, and start chowing down.

- **Allows you to get creative with your meals** - Finally, meal prepping allows you to get creative when it comes to your meals. The more you practice meal prepping, the more you'll learn how to cook healthy, tasty, keto-friendly dishes for your own enjoyment. This is also a way to keep you motivated to stick to your new diet.

Tips for Meal Planning

Meal planning is an important aspect of any new diet, not just keto. Although initially, it may seem overwhelming, it's actually a lot of fun once you commit to the process. To start off, you may need some basic kitchen tools in your keto cooking arsenal. These include the following items:

- Skillet

- High-quality chef's knife
- Blender or food processor
- Parchment paper
- Food containers (preferably made of glass)
- Vegetable spiralizer
- Kitchen scale

In Chapter 2, we went over the most basic keto-friendly ingredients. Combine those with these basic kitchen tools, and you'll be ready to go. Now, let's go over some tips to help you out:

- Plan your meals for the whole week. Set a schedule for your planning to sit down and lay out your meals and snacks for each day of the week. While doing this, have a separate sheet ready for your shopping list.

- Before you go shopping, check your pantry and refrigerator to see if you have any leftover meals or ingredients that you can use for the coming days or for the meals you have planned for the week. Then you can start crossing off items from your list.

- Once in a while, try to search for new recipes to include in your planned meals. Store your recipes in a folder on your computer or print them out and store them in a binder to use as a reference for your future meal planning.

- Before storing your meals in the refrigerator, make sure they are cooled completely. Also, plan your meals in such a way that you consume the ones that spoil easily first so you don't end up with food waste.

- Have fun with the process and with the meals you create. Don't take things too seriously. For instance, if you're not in the mood for the meal you had planned for that day, you may choose another one, or you may also choose to dine out with your friends occasionally and skip the meal you planned for the day. Just make sure that you carry over the leftover meals to the next week so you don't end up throwing them out.

Tips for Grocery Shopping

After planning your meals, it's time to start shopping. Again, it's helpful to check your pantry before you go shopping so you can start crossing out ingredients that you still have at home. Grocery shopping for the first time after you've decided to go keto is a different experience. You will have to be more aware of the foods you purchase to ensure that you only get ones that are keto-friendly.

The best way to do this is by checking the food labels of each item you pick up. In some supermarkets, they may have aisles that advertise these keto-friendly options, and some products may also have this same advertisement. In most cases, though, you will have to manually check food labels to ensure that you're getting the right products.

Don't worry - you won't have to spend so much time doing this for the rest of your life. As time goes by, you will get familiar with keto-friendly products from your local grocery stores. Just like when you used to pick out the same items that you loved back when you weren't keto, you'll also start picking out your own preferred keto-friendly products as time goes by.

Have you ever thought about what exactly should be on your grocery list? If you have no idea where to start, here are some ideas for your beginner, keto-friendly grocery list:

- High-quality meats, such as those that are grass-fed, pasture-raised, and wild-caught.
- Other protein sources that are soy-free, gluten-free, GMO-free, and dairy-free.
- Food sources that contain healthy fats, such as eggs, sardines, salmon, butter, cod liver oil, walnuts, hemp seeds, flax seeds, chia seeds, algae, and others.
- Keto-friendly sweeteners if you need them for your planned recipes.
- A lot of vegetables and fruits that are low in carbohydrates.

- Full-fat dairy products, such as heavy whipping cream, cheese, sour cream, and other products, which you can eat on their own or use in your recipes.
- Some ready-to-eat keto snacks so you always have something on-hand for when you get hungry at home or in the office.

Keeping Track of What You Eat and What You Like

These shopping and cooking tips will help make your keto journey easier and smoother. You won't have to rely on takeout, fast food, restaurants, and pre-packaged foods for your daily meals and snacks. You will save time and money and experience less stress. As time goes by, you will start learning more about what you like, and then you can plan your meals around your preferences to help keep you motivated, especially at the beginning.

Apart from keeping track of what you like, the more important thing is to record what you are eating. You should try to do this if you want to ensure the success of your keto journey. Some people keep a food journal as they start going keto. This is one of the best ways for you to monitor your daily food intake. If you don't want to keep a food journal, you can also keep all of your weekly meal plan lists in a clear book or binder and use it as your reference when you'd like to check what you have been eating.

If your main goal for following the keto diet is to lose weight, then you may want to keep track of your weight loss progress as well. Weigh yourself before you start your diet, and then set a date each month when you will measure your weight to check your progress. It's also ideal to check whether you've reached ketosis already or what level of ketosis you are currently in. To do this, you can either use ketone urine strips or you can invest in a blood ketone testing device, which is much more accurate.

It's important to get these things recorded so that you can make adjustments to your diet as needed. For instance, if you discover that you're not losing weight, you may check the portions of food you're consuming. Maybe you're eating too much or you might be eating foods that contain "hidden carbs". Also, keeping track of your progress allows you to determine whether you've already reached ketosis or not, which is the main goal of the keto diet, as you should know by now.

Chapter 6:
Keto and Weight Loss FAQ

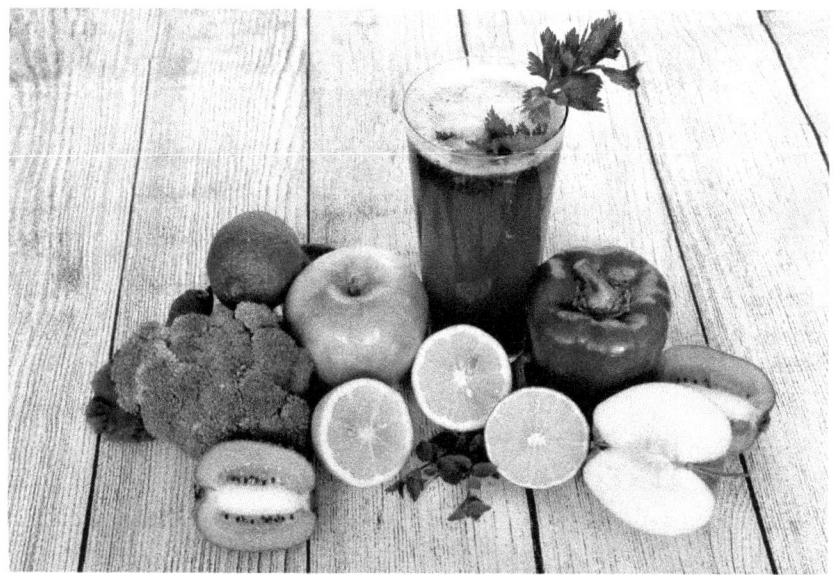

One of the most popular reasons why people choose to go keto is to lose weight. As a matter of fact, this is one of the most popular reasons that people choose to start any kind of diet. Whether you want to lose weight to have more confidence in yourself or you want to become healthier, going keto will be a huge advantage to you.

If your main reason for trying the diet is to lose weight, it's important for you to learn more about this benefit. In this chapter, we will be answering the most commonly asked questions concerning the keto diet and questions about the weight loss benefits of the diet.

FAQ About Keto

When you think about the basic principle behind the keto diet, you might not believe it right away. Imagine - you are eating a lot of fats in order for your body to burn fats more efficiently so you can lose weight. It may seem counterintuitive, but this is the foundation of the keto diet, and it's precisely why the diet is so effective.

To help you understand keto even more, let's take a look at the frequently asked questions about it below:

How many carbs should you eat on the keto diet?

If you want to achieve ketosis and enjoy all of the fat-burning benefits of this diet, it's important for you to restrict your intake of carbs. Depending on the type of keto diet you plan to follow, it's recommended that you eat fewer than 50 grams of carbs daily. However, if you choose one of the more restrictive types of keto diets, you might have to limit your intake to a mere 20 grams each day. Also, you may want to consider your age, activity level, biology, gender, and goals when trying to determine how many grams of carbs you should consume.

What is the keto flu?

The keto flu is one of the most common side effects of the keto diet and may develop as early as a couple of days after you've started your journey. If you start feeling a bit ill, this means that you may already have the keto flu. As long as you stay hydrated, get enough rest, and continue eating healthy foods, you will be able to overcome this condition. Apart from the keto flu, other common side effects may include a keto rash, diarrhea, and constipation, all of which are only temporary.

How do you know when you've achieved ketosis?

Being able to reach a state of ketosis varies greatly from one person to another. For some, it may take as little as a few days to reach this state while others have to wait for a couple of weeks. This depends on the ability of your body to adapt to fat-burning instead of burning glucose. As soon as you reach a state of ketosis, your body will naturally start producing ketones, and then you will notice that you have more energy, a reduction in your appetite, and improved focus. However, if you really want to know if you're in ketosis, you can use a blood or urine test.

Should you calculate your macros?

Macronutrients, or "macros", are the protein, fats, and carbs you eat in order to have energy. Although it's not a requirement to count and calculate your macros while following the keto diet, it is highly recommended that you do so. Calculating your macros allows you to learn more about the food you're eating and help you better understand the needs of your body.

Should you keep track of your net carbs?

If you want to keep track of anything, keep track of your net carbs. This refers to the carbs your body uses for fuel or energy. Recording this allows you to maintain ketosis by determining which foods to eat.

What should you do if you start experiencing constipation?

For a lot of people, starting a new diet may cause them to experience irregular bowel movements. This may happen when you start the keto diet as well. For this, there are some natural remedies that can help alleviate your constipation, including the following:

- Taking a magnesium supplement
- Drinking a lot of water
- Consuming 1 tablespoon of coconut oil
- Avoiding eating nuts for a while
- Consuming more high-fiber vegetables
- Consuming flax or chia seeds
- Drinking tea or coffee

Is it okay for you to drink alcohol while on the keto diet?

Alcoholic drinks aren't prohibited when you go keto. However, you must make sure that you choose what to drink wisely as a lot of alcoholic beverages may contain unnecessary sugar and carbs. If you really want to continue drinking alcohol, opt for clear liquor instead of those with flavors or drinks such as cocktails, which contain other ingredients.

FAQ About Weight Loss

Weight loss is one issue that a lot of people all over the globe are struggling with. It's so easy to get tempted by greasy, salty, sweet, and crunchy food, and yet we wonder why we find it to be so hard to shed those stubborn excess pounds. One of the major benefits of the keto diet is weight loss, which is exactly why so many people have chosen to go keto.

Let's review the most commonly asked questions about losing weight on the keto diet:

Is "dirty keto" a recommended variation of the keto diet?

Dirty keto is when you follow the same basic structure of the keto diet, but you don't restrict your consumption of fast foods, packaged foods, and processed foods. Although you may still be able to reach ketosis and start burning fat on this type of keto diet, you may also place yourself at risk for adverse side effects, such as weight gain and inflammation. Therefore, if you want to lose weight, this isn't the best choice for you.

Is it possible for you to eat too much fat?

Yes, it is entirely possible for you to eat too much fat. While following keto, you're recommended to consume high amounts of fat, but you still need to remain at a caloric deficit if you would like to lose weight. When you eat too much fat, it pushes you over the required caloric deficit, resulting in a caloric surplus. This is why it's recommended to count your macros to make sure that you're getting the right amount to make the diet effective.

Will the keto diet spike your cholesterol?

Consuming more saturated fats may elevate your total cholesterol, your good cholesterol, and sometimes even your bad cholesterol. However, if you're only consuming high-quality, healthy fats, this is a good thing, so you needn't worry about it.

How much weight will you lose on the keto diet?

The answer to this question varies from person to person. For instance, if you follow the keto diet and pair it with regular exercise, there's a higher chance that you will lose more weight compared to someone who simply follows the diet but continues having a sedentary lifestyle. If you really want to lose a lot of weight on keto, make sure to follow the diet properly and consider pairing it with another type of healthy diet or additional healthy habits.

Why aren't you losing weight on keto?

There are several reasons why one will not lose weight, even after following the keto diet for a long time. They may not be eating enough, eating too much, or they might even be eating the wrong types of foods. So, if you discover that you're not losing weight, you may have to make a few adjustments to your diet.

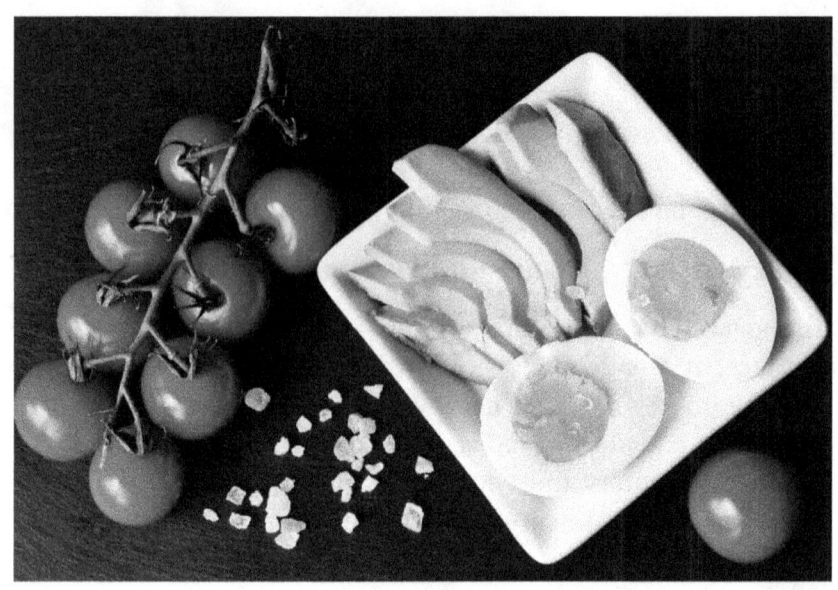
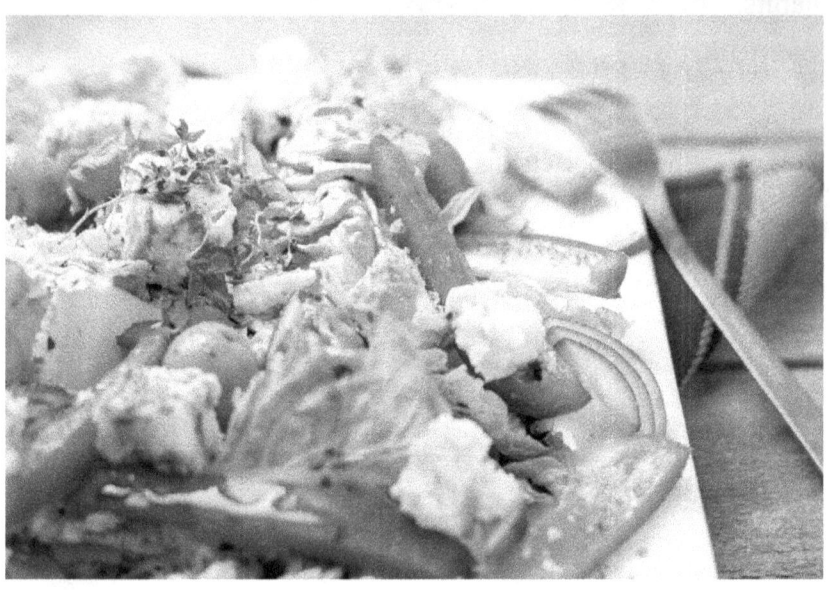

Chapter 7:
Sample Meal Plan

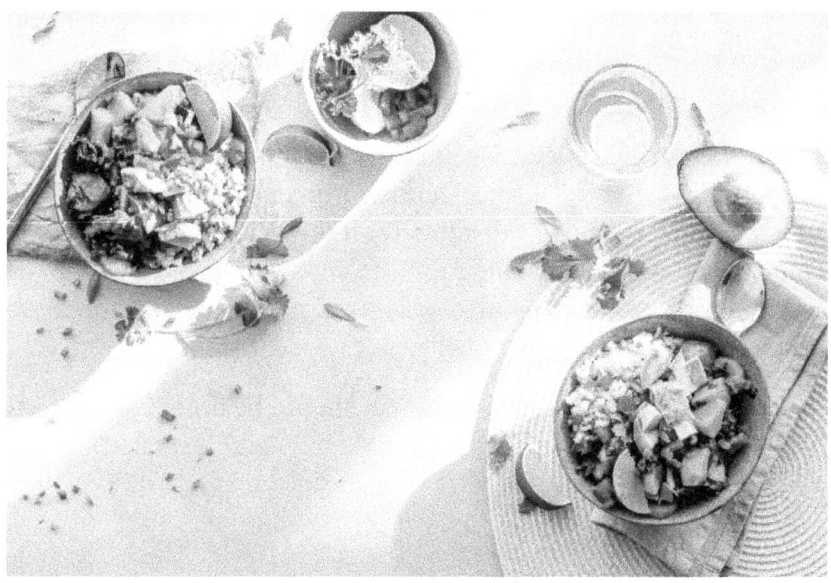

You now have all the basic information you need to start your keto journey. Learning all about the keto diet is an important aspect of beginning to use it. We've covered the definition of the diet, what it entails, how you can get started, and some tips and strategies to help you out. From knowing the dos and don'ts to learning all about cooking and shopping, you are now armed with a great deal of valuable information that can help you take the challenging first step into going keto.

So what else is there for you to learn? As a bonus for you, we will go through a sample meal plan. This chapter is all about food. We've covered how the keto diet is quite restrictive since you need to avoid a number of foods while only consuming certain types of foods. Creating your own meal plan is very important when you start and attempt to maintain this diet.

Even though the diet is quite popular, you won't really find keto-friendly options everywhere. Some restaurants and supermarkets may offer keto-friendly fares, but if you're unlucky enough to live in a place where keto hasn't caught on, you can easily get derailed. When this happens, you might go right back to your unhealthy eating habits, thus wasting all the time and effort you spent learning about and initiating your diet.

One-Day Sample Meal Plan

If you have never tried planning your meals before, you should keep in mind that it does take some getting used to. You will have to start training yourself to actually sit down and take the time to think about what you will be eating each day for a whole week. The learning process does involve some trial and error, but the more you practice, the better you will get at it.

To give you a better idea of what you should be doing, take a look at this sample meal plan for one whole day (with explanations for some of them that you don't need to include while you're planning):

Breakfast

- **Option 1:** Mushroom, feta, and spinach omelet paired with keto coffee.
  You can add fat to your coffee by using butter, bone broth protein, or MCT oil.
  This is an excellent breakfast combination that contains healthy fats and protein. It will keep you full and help curb your midmorning cravings.
- **Option 2:** Unsweetened yogurt with chia seeds, walnuts, a handful of raspberries, and full-fat sour cream paired with whole milk.
  If you choose to use this combination for breakfast, make sure to count the carbs and consume the proper portion. All types of yogurts naturally contain lactose, which is a kind of carb.
  You can also pair this with a protein that's free of carbs, such as two eggs, to balance out your macros.

Lunch

- **Option 1:** Oven-cooked salmon with broccoli.
  This healthy combination features a great source of healthy fats along with a high-fiber, low-carb vegetable.
- **Option 2:** A healthy salad containing avocado, bacon, spiced pumpkin seeds, cheese, and a couple of grape tomatoes paired with blue cheese, ranch, or another type of salad dressing that's high in fat.
- **Option 3:** A keto-friendly "lunchable" containing nitrate-free ham, grilled chicken, pickle slices, a boiled egg, cheese cubes, a couple of grape tomatoes, broccoli or cauliflower, a handful of almonds or walnuts, ranch dressing, and guacamole.

Dinner

- **Option 1:** Keto-friendly Caesar salad with bacon, chicken breast, romaine lettuce, and parmesan.
  This salad is super filling since it's high in protein. To add fat to your salad, pair it with a lot of cheese and a tasty olive-oil dressing.
- **Option 2:** Sautéed ground beef (grass fed) with low-carb tomato sauce and onions. Pair this with low-carb shirataki or zucchini noodles.
  Again, you can add fat to this meal by sautéing the noodles in either garlic-infused oil or olive oil.
- **Option 3:** Grilled chicken, yellow squash, zucchini, and eggplant paired with tomatoes that have been sautéed with olive oil and garlic.
  To add more fat, create a sauce using coconut cream or heavy cream to help balance out your macros.

Snacks

- **Option 1:** Modified BLT roll-ups using avocado and turkey.
  This is an excellent combination of protein and fat to fill you up until your next meal.

- **Option 2:** Create a cucumber and cream cheese sandwich using the cucumber slices as the bread.
  This snack is tasty, refreshing, low-carb, and highly satisfying.
- **Option 3:** Raw slices of zucchini paired with spicy guacamole.

Foods to Eat

As you can see, when you plan your meals, it's important to be as specific as possible, especially during your first few weeks or months of planning. If you really want to be precise, you can do research on the macro or nutrient content of each ingredient you're using. In fact, there are even some recipes out there that provide the exact nutrient content information. These recipes are very useful, especially when you aren't that familiar with counting or calculating your macros yet.

As you learn, you can start off by using recipes that already include with the information you need so you don't have to spend too much time figuring out the nutrient content. Eventually, you will learn how to calculate your macros more effectively, and this is when you can determine the numbers on your own. When planning your meals, you should have a good idea of what kinds of foods actually fit into your diet. To guide you, here are the foods you can eat on the keto diet:

Fats and Oils

When you go keto, your daily diet must consist of mostly fats. You can combine these fat sources in a variety of ways, like in making dressings, sauces, or by simply drizzling them over your meals. Our bodies need fats in order to function, especially when you're planning to go keto. However, you shouldn't eat just any types of fats and oils, as there are some that are considered to be unhealthy. Here's a short overview for you when it comes to fats:

- **Saturated fats:** These include coconut oil, butter, lard, ghee, and others. These are healthy types of fats that you can include in your diet.

- **Monounsaturated fats:** These fats include avocado oil, macadamia oil, olive oil, and others. These are also healthy types of fats that you can include in your diet.
- **Polyunsaturated fats:** The naturally occurring varieties can be found in fatty fish and animal protein, and these are good for you. However, the processed varieties aren't.
- **Trans fats:** These are chemically-altered processed fats that you must avoid at all costs, especially if you want to lose weight or avoid developing heart disease.

Protein

When it comes to protein, it's best to opt for the grass-fed and pasture-raised varieties as these will minimize your steroid hormone and bacteria intake. Also, it's more recommended to choose dark meat when possible, as it is fattier than white meat. Fish is also an excellent source of protein since it also contains healthy omega-3s.

In terms of red meat, the only types you might have to avoid are cured and processed varieties, as these may contain added sugars and other unnecessary ingredients. If you enjoy steak, choose the fattier cuts.

One thing to remember in terms of protein is that you should only stick with moderate amounts. Eating excess meat might decrease your ketone production while increasing your glucose production. While on keto, your goal must be nutritional ketosis, which means that you should consume the proper amounts and ratios of macros.

Vegetables and Fruit

Almost all kinds of diets would recommend that you increase your intake of vegetables and fruits. This applies to the keto diet as well. However, there are also some types of fruits and veggies that you must avoid as they contain high amounts of carbs and sugar.

The best possible kinds of veggies for the keto diet include those that are dark, green, and leafy; these are the ones that contain high amounts of nutrients and low amounts of carbs. In terms of fruits, only choose ones that aren't high in carbs and sugar. When it comes to fruits and veggies, both fresh and frozen varieties are okay.

Dairy Products

Dairy products are usually paired with keto meals, but you should be very mindful when it comes to these types of foods. If you really want to include dairy in your diet, opt for the organic and raw varieties. Also, choose full-fat products instead of low-fat or fat-free ones, as these are more filling and contain more fat.

Nuts and Seeds

It's best to consume nuts and seeds that have been roasted, as this process eliminates any anti-nutrients. You can add raw nuts to your meal for extra texture and flavor. You may also choose to snack on these by themselves, but don't do this too frequently, as this might slow down your weight loss. Also, some nuts do contain a fair amount of carbs, so make sure to choose your nuts wisely.

Water and Beverages

Water is a definite yes on the keto diet. In fact, you should drink a lot of water to avoid getting dehydrated as you start your new diet. For other types of beverages, it's okay to drink coffee, tea, and any other beverages that don't contain added sugars.

Foods to Avoid

Now comes the hard part; in this section, we will cover the foods that you must avoid. Since you have a primary goal to reach a state of ketosis while following the keto diet, it's important for you to choose the foods you eat wisely. For one, be careful of certain foods that may contain hidden carbs. Some common examples of these include the following:

- **Low-carb food items** such as snacks, bars, and other foods. If you want to opt for these options, make sure to check the labels first.

- **Spices** such as ginger, cinnamon, onion powder, garlic powder may contain more carbs.
- **Berries and fruits** may contain high amounts of sugar. If you don't want to eliminate these from your diet, make sure to control your portion sizes.
- **Tomato-based products** such as canned tomatoes or tomato sauces can be bad for your diet. Make sure you check the labels of such products as some companies may modify the recommended serving sizes to make consumers believe that these are the "healthier" options.
- **Condiments** may contain added carbs and sugars, so you should check both the nutrition and ingredient lists.
- **Chilis and peppers** may contain carbs and sugars, so choose them carefully.
- **Diet soda** may contain sugars. Even if you can drink these sodas while you're on the keto diet, it's recommended to avoid them completely, as they contain artificial sweeteners.
- **Chocolate** is also allowed on keto, but you should control your portions carefully. Also, you may want to choose dark chocolate which contains fewer carbs (the darker, the better).
- **Medications** should be taken with caution. There are a lot of flu remedies, cold medications, and cough syrups that contain high amounts of sugar. If ever you get sick while on this diet, you can opt for diabetic or sugar-free alternatives of these medications.

These are just some examples of foods that may contain hidden carbs and sugars, but there are also some food items that you must avoid completely while you're on keto. When planning your meals, make sure to stay away from the following foods:

- **Sugar**, including food items that are high in sugar, such as sports drinks, candies, ice cream, juices, and more.
- **Grains**, which are found in wheat products, cakes, corn, rice, beer, cereals, and so on.

- **Starch**, which can be found in muesli, oats, and even some types of fruits and vegetables.
- **Low-fat products** tend to contain higher amounts of sugar and carbs compared to their full-fat counterparts.

Generally, it's more recommended to choose "real foods" over processed foods as you can be more certain about their nutrient and macro content. However, if you do choose any processed foods, don't forget to check the labels to ensure that they're keto-friendly.

Conclusion:
Starting Your Keto Journey

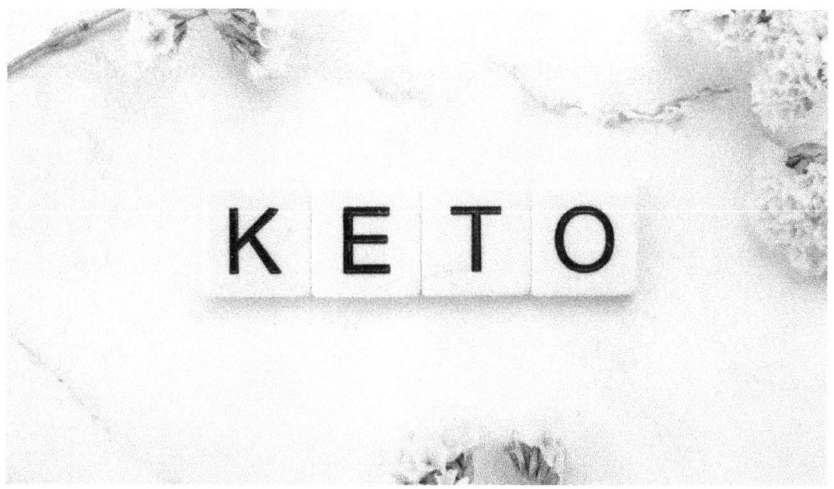

There you have it - all the fundamental information you need to start your keto journey. Although this is one of the best and most beneficial diets out there, it's not recommended for everyone. Before you start on this diet, make sure that you know exactly what you're getting yourself into. Whether you're at the peak of your health or suffering from a medical condition, it's best to speak with your doctor about any diet and lifestyle changes you plan to undertake.

Once you are given the go-ahead by your physician, it's time to start planning. Try to remember everything we have gone through from the start of this book all the way to the last chapter. You've already taken one of the first and most important steps, which is to learn everything that you can about the keto diet. Now it's time to start setting your goals and planning the steps you will take at the beginning of your journey.

Just remember to make health and safety your main priority. Never push yourself too hard, and if you slip up, forgive yourself for it. Going keto is a huge change, especially if it's your first time trying to follow a structured, healthy diet. You can make things a lot easier by adopting a positive attitude toward the diet. Think of it as an investment in yourself. When you encounter any challenges, find ways to overcome them without giving up. Motivate yourself externally and internally to ensure that you stick with your diet no matter what. In time, you'll start experiencing the many benefits and understand that you are living a happier and healthier life.

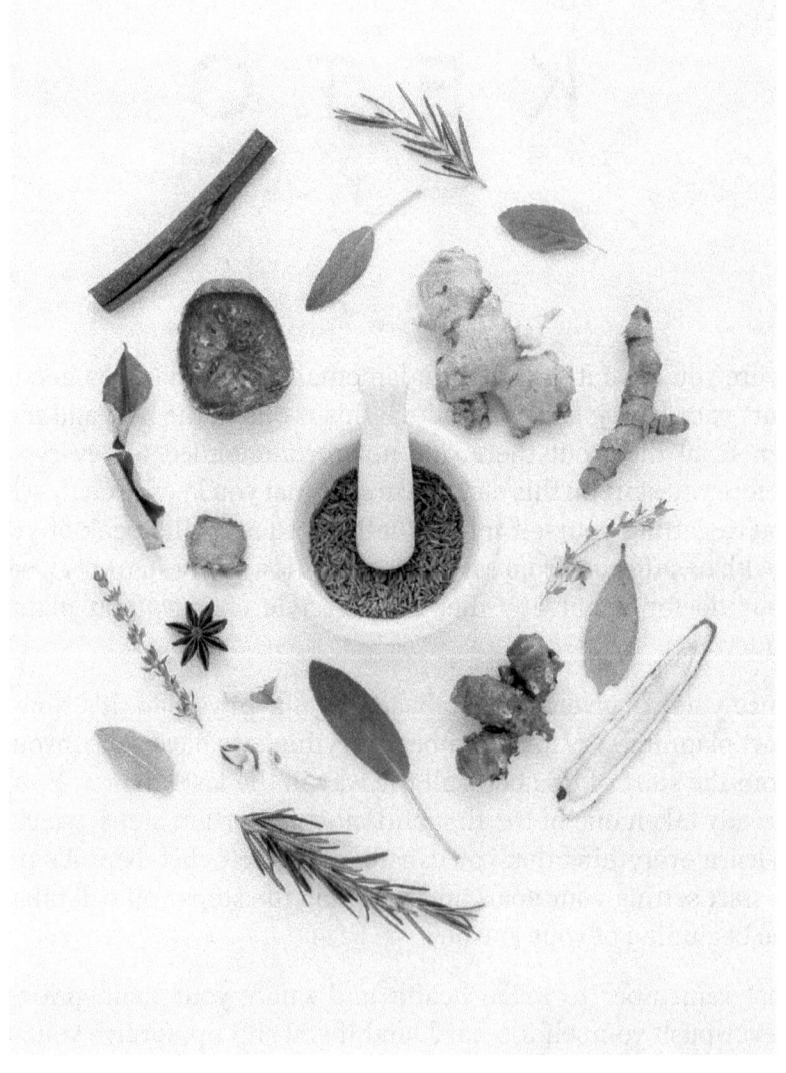

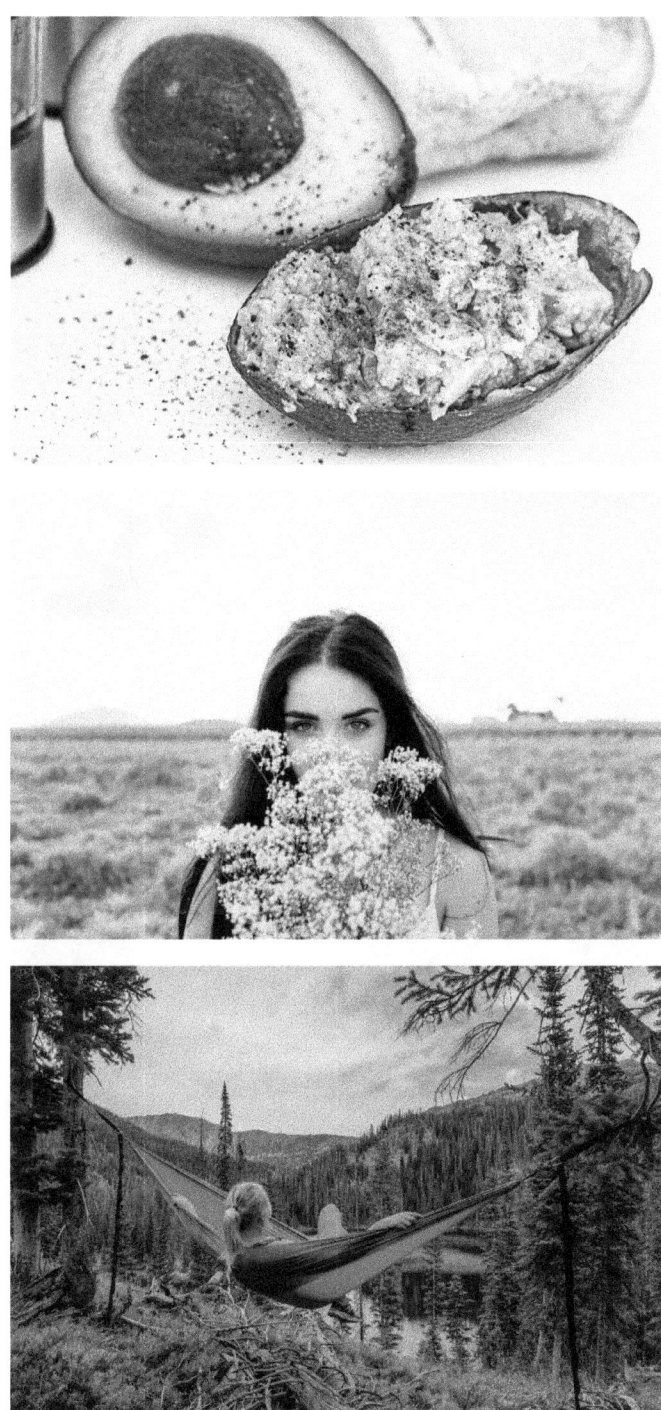

References

5 Steps to Transition into a Keto Diet | Ruled Me. (2019). Retrieved from https://www.ruled.me/transition-to-keto-diet/

9 Proven Benefits of a Ketogenic Diet - DrJockers.com. (2019). Retrieved from https://drjockers.com/benefits-ketogenic-diet/

Axe, J. Keto Diet For Beginners Made Easy: The Ultimate Guide to "Keto". (2019). Retrieved from https://draxe.com/guide-to-keto-diet-for-beginners/

Beginner Keto Grocery List. (2018). Retrieved from https://theketoqueens.com/beginner-keto-grocery-list/?cn-reloaded=1

Bowman, R., & Bohl, M. Do's and Don'ts on the Keto Diet. (2019). Retrieved from https://www.doctoroz.com/article/do-s-and-don-ts-keto-diet

Cudmore, D. Should You Combine A Ketogenic Diet With Paleo?. (2019). Retrieved from https://blog.paleohacks.com/ketogenic-diet-and-paleo/#

Easter, M. Inside the Rise of Keto: How an Extreme Diet Went Mainstream. (2019). Retrieved from https://www.menshealth.com/nutrition/a25775330/keto-diet-history/

Eliason, N. Easy Keto: How to Sustain a Ketogenic Diet with 5 Simple Rules - Nat Eliason. (2019). Retrieved from https://www.nateliason.com/blog/easy-keto

Gordon, B. What is the Ketogenic Diet. (2019). Retrieved from https://www.eatright.org/health/weight-loss/fad-diets/what-is-the-ketogenic-diet

Gustin, A. Keto Diet For Beginners: 5 Easy Steps To Get Started - Perfect Keto. (2019). Retrieved from https://perfectketo.com/keto-diet-for-beginners/

Holland, K. The 10 Foods You Should Buy to Build Your Keto Pantry. (2018). Retrieved from https://www.myrecipes.com/ingredients/essential-keto-diet-foods

How to Create Effective, Simple and SMART Ketogenic Diet Goals. (2017). Retrieved from https://centsibleketo.com/how-to-create-effective-simple-and-smart-ketogenic-diet-goals/

How To Start a Keto Diet: The Ultimate Guide. (2019). Retrieved from https://perfectketo.com/guide/ultimate-start-guide-ketogenic-diet/

Hyman, M. What Is the Keto Diet (and Should You Try It)?. (2018). Retrieved from https://health.clevelandclinic.org/what-is-the-keto-diet-and-should-you-try-it/

Intermittent Fasting and Keto: Should You Combine the Two?. (2019). Retrieved from https://www.healthline.com/nutrition/intermittent-fasting-and-keto#benefits

Kernaghan, C. My Keto Journey. (2018). Retrieved from https://medium.com/@chriskernaghan/my-keto-journey-90fca024007

Keto Diet Do's and Don'ts - What I Need to Remember While Eating Keto. (2019). Retrieved from http://ketogenicdietforwomen.com/keto-diet-dos-and-donts/

Keto Diet Plan: Dos and Don'ts - Brown Apron. (2017). Retrieved from https://brownapron.com/blog/blogs/keto-diet-plan-dos-donts/

Keto Diet Plan For Beginners: Everything You Need To Know Before Starting. (2019). Retrieved from https://keto-mojo.com/pages/keto-diet-plan

Keto FAQ: Everything You Ever Wanted to Know About the Keto Diet. (2019). Retrieved from https://blog.bulletproof.com/keto-faq/

Ketogenic Diet FAQ | Ruled Me. (2019). Retrieved from https://www.ruled.me/ketogenic-diet-faq/

Ketogenic Diet Food List: Everything You Need to Know | Ruled Me. (2019). Retrieved from https://www.ruled.me/ketogenic-diet-food-list/

Lipman, F. Time to Go Keto? 6 Thoughts on the Ketogenic Diet - Be Well. (2018). Retrieved from https://www.bewell.com/blog/6-thoughts-ketogenic-diet/

Livingston, M. 8 tricks for doing the keto diet without driving yourself crazy. (2018). Retrieved from https://www.businessinsider.com/8-tricks-that-help-with-keto-diet-2018-7

Malacoff, J. The Keto Meal Plan for Beginners. (2019). Retrieved from https://www.shape.com/weight-loss/tips-plans/keto-meal-plan-beginners-high-fat-diet

Occhipinti, M. What is the History and Evolution of the Keto Diet?. (2018). Retrieved from https://www.afpafitness.com/blog/what-is-the-history-and-evolution-of-the-keto-diet

Our 10 Favorite Keto Success Stories of 2019. (2019). Retrieved from https://www.ketogenicsupplementreviews.com/blog/keto-success-stories/

Roberts, M. Keto Do's and Don'ts. (2019). Retrieved from https://www.ketovangelist.com/keto-dos-and-donts/

The Beginner's Guide To Meal Planning On Keto In 4 Simple Steps. (2019). Retrieved from https://missfitliving.com/keto-meal-planning/

The Easiest Way to Track Carbs on a Keto Diet | Ruled Me. (2019). Retrieved from https://www.ruled.me/carb-tracking-for-keto-diet/

The Essential Guide to Effortless Keto Meal Prep - Perfect Keto. (2018). Retrieved from https://perfectketo.com/keto-meal-prep/

Wells, K. How to Meal Plan - The Ultimate Guide to Meal Planning | Wellness Mama. (2019). Retrieved from https://wellnessmama.com/5345/meal-planning/

https://www.healthline.com/nutrition/ketogenic-diet-101#diet-types

www.ingramcontent.com/pod-product-compliance
Lightning Source LLC
Chambersburg PA
CBHW071124030426
42336CB00013BA/2200